Sandeep Kumar Panigrahi

Single oral dose medication of Albendazole & DEC in Filariasis

Diptirani Rath
Sandeep Kumar Panigrahi

Single oral dose medication of Albendazole & DEC in Filariasis

A study on the safety and acceptability of single high dose of Albendazole with DEC in Microfilariaemic individuals

LAP LAMBERT Academic Publishing

Impressum/Imprint (nur für Deutschland/only for Germany)
Bibliografische Information der Deutschen Nationalbibliothek: Die Deutsche Nationalbibliothek verzeichnet diese Publikation in der Deutschen Nationalbibliografie; detaillierte bibliografische Daten sind im Internet über http://dnb.d-nb.de abrufbar.
Alle in diesem Buch genannten Marken und Produktnamen unterliegen warenzeichen-, marken- oder patentrechtlichem Schutz bzw. sind Warenzeichen oder eingetragene Warenzeichen der jeweiligen Inhaber. Die Wiedergabe von Marken, Produktnamen, Gebrauchsnamen, Handelsnamen, Warenbezeichnungen u.s.w. in diesem Werk berechtigt auch ohne besondere Kennzeichnung nicht zu der Annahme, dass solche Namen im Sinne der Warenzeichen- und Markenschutzgesetzgebung als frei zu betrachten wären und daher von jedermann benutzt werden dürften.

Coverbild: www.ingimage.com

Verlag: LAP LAMBERT Academic Publishing GmbH & Co. KG
Heinrich-Böcking-Str. 6-8, 66121 Saarbrücken, Deutschland
Telefon +49 681 3720-310, Telefax +49 681 3720-3109
Email: info@lap-publishing.com

Approved by: Rourkela, BPUT, Diss., 2010

Herstellung in Deutschland:
Schaltungsdienst Lange o.H.G., Berlin
Books on Demand GmbH, Norderstedt
Reha GmbH, Saarbrücken
Amazon Distribution GmbH, Leipzig
ISBN: 978-3-8465-8029-5

Imprint (only for USA, GB)
Bibliographic information published by the Deutsche Nationalbibliothek: The Deutsche Nationalbibliothek lists this publication in the Deutsche Nationalbibliografie; detailed bibliographic data are available in the Internet at http://dnb.d-nb.de.
Any brand names and product names mentioned in this book are subject to trademark, brand or patent protection and are trademarks or registered trademarks of their respective holders. The use of brand names, product names, common names, trade names, product descriptions etc. even without a particular marking in this works is in no way to be construed to mean that such names may be regarded as unrestricted in respect of trademark and brand protection legislation and could thus be used by anyone.

Cover image: www.ingimage.com

Publisher: LAP LAMBERT Academic Publishing GmbH & Co. KG
Heinrich-Böcking-Str. 6-8, 66121 Saarbrücken, Germany
Phone +49 681 3720-310, Fax +49 681 3720-3109
Email: info@lap-publishing.com

Printed in the U.S.A.
Printed in the U.K. by (see last page)
ISBN: 978-3-8465-8029-5

Acknowledgement

It is a great opportunity for me to convey my thanks through this small piece of acknowledgement to those precious persons without whose help, assistance and guidance this piece of work would have been impossible to complete.

I sincerely thanks my husband **Dr Sandeep Kumar Panigrahi**, for his helping hand for preparing and finalizing this book based on my thesis.

I hereby place on record with utmost sincerity, my esteemed and profound sense of gratitude to **Dr B. Dwivedi**, of RMRC (Bhubaneswar) for his constant supervision, valuable guidance and advice in the course of my dissertation work and the preparation of this thesis.

I would like to convey my sincere thanks to **Dr. P. N. Murthy**, Principal and Director of Royal College of Pharmacy and Health Sciences to give me scope and provide facilities to learn and explore to my full potentials in the field of Pharmacology.

I express my deep sense of gratitude to **Dr. S. K. Kar**, Director, Regional Medical Research centre, Bhubaneswar for giving me the opportunity to carry out my project work in this reputed institution.

I would also like to thank my teachers at RCPHS who have always supported and showered their wisdom on me. Not to forget the contribution of my friends and my parents for constantly supporting me throughout the research work.

Last but not the least, I would also like to place on record contribution of laboratory animals who sacrificed their life for the human beings.

Diptirani Rath

MPharm (Pharmacology)

This page has been intentionally left blank

CONTENTS

Sl. No.	Topic	Page No
1	Introduction	1
2	Aims and Objectives	21
3	Literature review	22
4	Study in Microfilaraemic Individuals	
	i. Study design and methods	30
	ii. Results	36
5	Study in albino mice	
	i. Study design and methods	41
	ii. Results	45
6	Discussion	49
7	Conclusion	50
	References	51

This page has been intentionally left blank

List of tables

Sl. No	Name of table	Page no
1.1	Differences between W. bancroftii & B. malayi	4
1.2	Agent factor	10
4.1	Baseline parameters of enrolled subjects	37
4.2	Post drug evaluation	38
4.3	Adverse events	38
4.4	Mf count at baseline and follow up after 6 months	39
5.1	Drug treatment protocol	43
5.2	Signs of acute toxicity	45
5.3	Clinical signs of acute toxicity	46
5.4	Individual body weights	47
5.5	Hematological parameters in study animals	47
5.6	Clinical biochemistry	48
5.7	Necropsy and organ weights	48

List of figures

Sl. No	Figure	Page no
1	Life cycle of W. bancroftii	6
2	Microfilaria {Male (short) and female (long)}	7
3	Microscopic examination of the blood smear	7
4	Elephantiasis of leg	7

List of abbreviations

AE	Adverse Event
ALB	Albendazole
CRF	Case report form
CR	Creatinine
DEC	Di-ethyl Carbamazine
DNA	Deoxy Ribonucleic Acid
ELISA	Enzyme Linked Immunosorbant Assay
FDS	Filarial Dance Sign
GCP	Good Clinical Practice
GSK	Glaxo Smith Kline
HDLs	High Density Lipoproteins
ICH	International Conference on Harmonization
ICMR	Indian Council of Medical Research
ICT	Immuno-chromatographic Card Test
IRB	Institutional Review Board
KIMS	Kalinga Institute of Medical Sciences
LDLs	Low density lipoproteins
LF	Lymphatic Filariasis
MDT	Mass Drug Treatment
Mf	Microfilaria
RMRC	Regional Medical Research Centre
SAE	Serious Adverse Event
Wb	*Wuchereria bancroftii*
Hb	Hemoglobin
VLDLs	Very Low Density Lipoprotein
WHO	World Health Organization

INTRODUCTION

Filariasis has been a major public health problem in India. The disease was recorded in India as early as 6th century B.C. by the famous Indian physician, Susruta in his book 'Susruta Samhita'. National Filaria Control Programme (NFCP) was launched in the country in 1955 with the objective of delimiting the problem and to undertake control measures in endemic areas. The manifold increase in filariasis during last four decades reflects failure of filariasis control programs. Currently there may be up to 31 million microfilaraemics, 23 million cases of symptomatic filariasis, and about 473 million individuals potentially at risk of infection in the country. Lymphatic filariasis (LF) is a major impediment to socioeconomic development and is responsible for immense psychosocial suffering among the affected.

Filariasis is a parasitic and infectious disease that is caused by thread-like filarial nematode worms. Filarial nematodes which use humans as the definitive host are divided into 3 groups according to the niche within the body that they occupy and they cause diseases like Lymphatic Filariasis, Subcutaneous Filariasis, and Serous Cavity Filariasis. Lymphatic Filariasis is caused by the worms Wuchereria bancrofti, Brugia malayi, and Brugia timori. These worms occupy the lymphatic system, including the lymph nodes and in chronic cases these worms lead to the disease Elephantiasis.

Individuals infected by filarial worms may be described as either "microfilaraemic" or "amicrofilaraemic," depending on whether or not microfilaria is found in their peripheral blood. Filariasis is diagnosed in microfilaraemic cases primarily through direct observation of microfilaria in the peripheral blood. Lymphatic filariasis is caused by infection with one of three nematodes, Wuchereria bancrofti, Brugia malayi, or Brugia timori. These agents cause similar clinical syndromes. They are a major cause of disfigurement and disability in endemic areas, leading to significant economic and psychosocial impact. All three parasites have basically similar life cycles; in man. Adult worms live in the lymphatic vessels while their offspring, the microfilariae circulate in the peripheral blood and are available to the infect mosquito vectors when they come for a blood meal. The disease manifestations range from none to both acute and chronic manifestations such as lymphangitis, lymphadenitis, and elephantiasis of genitals, legs and arms or as a sensitivity state such as Tropical pulmonary eosinophilia or as atypical form such as filarial arthritis[14].

Though not fatal, the disease is responsible for considerable suffering, deformity and disability.

1

HISTORY:

Lymphatic Filariasis is thought to have affected humans since approximately 4000 years ago. Artifacts from ancient Egypt (2000 BC) and the Nok civilization in West Africa (500 BC) show possible elephantiasis symptoms. The first clear reference to the disease occurs in ancient Greek literature, where scholars differentiated the often similar symptoms of lymphatic filariasis from those of leprosy. The first documentation of symptoms occurred in the 16th century, when Jan Huyghen van Linschoten wrote about the disease during the exploration of Goa. Similar symptoms were reported by subsequent explorers in areas of Asia and Africa, though an understanding of the disease did not began to develop until centuries later.

In 1866, Timothy Lewis, building on the work of Jean-Nicolas Demarquay and Otto Henry Wucherer, made the connection between microfilariae and elephantiasis, establishing the course of research that would ultimately explain the disease. In 1876, Joseph Bancroft discovered the adult form of the worm. In 1877, the life cycle involving an arthropod vector was theorized by Patrick Manson, who proceeded to demonstrate the presence of the worms in mosquitoes. Manson incorrectly hypothesized that the disease was transmitted through skin contact with water in which the mosquitoes had laid eggs. In 1900, George Carmichael Low determined the actual transmission method by discovering the presence of the worm in the proboscis of the mosquito vector.

AREAS AFFECTED:

Filariasis is a global health problem. It is a major social and economic trouble in the tropics and subtropics of Africa, Asia, and some parts f Americas affecting over 120 million people in 80 counties. *Wuchereria bancrofti* is the most widespread of the human filariae in the world. The majority of infections occur in Asia, but this parasite also causes considerable problems in Africa and the north-west of South America. In India, it is distributed chiefly along the sea coast and the banks of big rivers. The disease is endemic all over India, except Jammu and Kashmir, Himachal Pradesh, Punjab, Haryana, Delhi, Chandigarh, Sikkim, Tripura, Arunachal Pradesh and Mizoram. But; recently it has also been reported in Punjab, Rajasthan and Delhi.

Present estimates indicate that about 467 million people are living in zones where Lymphatic Filariasis is endemic, of which; 109 million are living in urban areas and the rest in rural areas. There are estimated to be at least 6 million attacks of acute filariasis per year, and at

2

least 20 million persons currently have one or more chronic filarial lesions. It is estimated that more than 120 million people worldwide are infected with one of these three microfilariae. More than 90 percent of these infections are due to W. bancrofti, and the remainders are mostly due to B. malayi. Estimates suggest that more than 40 million infected individuals are seriously incapacitated and disfigured by the disease. A study from India, which accounts for 40 percent of the global prevalence of infection, estimated that a minimum of $842 million is lost each year there, secondary to treatment costs and working days lost from filariasis. Another Indian study suggested that patients with chronic filariasis lose around 29 days of work per year due to complications of infection, highlighting the considerable burden the disease places on individuals and on the community. Adult worms are gradually acquired over years, slowly accumulating and producing microfilariae in infected individuals. Thus, the prevalence of microfilaremia in endemic communities increases with age. After the third or fourth decade of life, most people have been exposed and the proportion of infected individuals remains relatively constant. Nations found to be endemic tend to be tropical or subtropical due to the optimal habitat for the vectors of lymphatic filariasis. Ambient humidity is also necessary for the survival of the infective larva stage of the microfilariae. Populations at high risk for contracting or developing a lymphatic filariasis infection are primarily poor, and a majority of the cases are concentrated in rural areas. Lymphatic filariasis is often associated with areas that have poor sanitation and housing quality Poorer, rural communities are also typically built around optimal environments for vectors, including marshes or rivers, and tend to lack the resources or capabilities to control for vectors, and transmission is high as a result.

Although there is an established high prevalence of transmission in rural areas of endemic areas, little research has been done around urban transmission of endemic areas. Although the WHO estimated a low occurrence of less than 1% of urban cases of lymphatic filariasis resulting from urban transmission, this study revealed that approximately 6% of urban cases of lymphatic filariasis were results of urban transmission. According to the authors of this study, and other members of the public health community, this percentage is high enough to confirm transmission of lymphatic filariasis in urban areas. As a result of this study, a Mass Drug Treatment (MDT) program has been installed in the urban areas of the study, and urban treatment programs such as this are spreading throughout endemic regions.

3

Table: 1.1 Differences between Mf of W. bancrofti and B. malayi

Features	Mf of *W. bancrofti*	Mf of *B. malayi*
General appearance	Graceful, sweeping curves	Crinkled, secondary curves
Length	244-296 µm	177-230 µm
Free cephalic space	As long as broad	Nearly twice as long as broad
Excretory Pore	Not prominent	Prominent
Caudal end	Uniformly tapering to a delicate point, No terminal nuclei present	Kinkled and two terminal nuclei present
Nuclear column	Nuclei discrete	Smudged

PERIODICITY:

The mf of *W. bancrofti* and *B. malayi* occurring in India displays a nocturnal periodicity, i.e. they appear in large numbers at night and retreat from the blood stream during the day. This is a biological adaptation to the nocturnal biting habits of the vector mosquitoes. The cues used by the mosquitoes to regulate their periodicity appear to be physiological signals from the host such as oxygen tension in the blood and body temperature. The maximum density of Mf in blood is reported between 10pm and 2 am. When the sleeping habits of hosts are altered, reversal in periodicity has been observed.

LIFE CYCLE:

During a blood meal, an infected mosquito introduces third-stage filarial larvae onto the skin of the human host, where they penetrate into the bite wound (Fig: 1)

❶. They develop in adults that commonly reside in the lymphatic

❷. The female worms measure 80 to 100 mm in length and 0.24 to 0.30 mm in diameter, while the males measure about 40 mm by .1 mm. Adults produce microfilariae measuring 244 to 296 µm by 7.5 to 10 µm, which are sheathed and have nocturnal periodicity, except the South Pacific microfilariae which have the absence of marked periodicity. The microfilariae migrate into lymph and blood channels moving actively through lymph and blood

❸. A mosquito ingests the microfilariae during a blood meal

❹. After ingestion, the microfilariae lose their sheaths and some of them work their way through the wall of the proventriculus and cardiac portion of the mosquito's midgut and reach the thoracic muscles

❺. There microfilariae develop into first-stage larvae

4

❻ And subsequently into third-stage infective larvae

❼ The third-stage infective larvae migrate through the hemocoel to the mosquito's prosbocis

❽ And can infect another human when the mosquito takes a blood meal

The following stages of development takes place in the vector:-

A. Unsheathing: The larva comes out of its sheath within 2 hours of its ingestion. This takes place in the stomach of the mosquito.

B. First stage larva: After unsheathing the larva is able to penetrate the stomach wall of the mosquito which it does in 6-12 hours and migrate to the thoracic muscles where it grows and develops into a sausage shaped (short thick) form.

C. Second stage larva: The larva molts and increases in length (long thick form) with the development of an alimentary canal, but is relatively inactive.

D. Third stage larva: There is a final molt to the third stage or infective larva (long thin form) which may be found in any part of the insect. It is highly active or motile. When it migrates to the proboscis of the mosquito, it is ready to be transmitted to a new hit and the mosquito is said to be infective. Under optimum conditions of temperature and humidity, the duration of mosquito cycle (extrinsic incubation period) is between 10-14 days. In the human host, the infective larvae develop into adult male and female worms.

The worms are 0.2 mm wide and can be up to 10 cm long. (Fig: 2)

- Male→2.5-4cm(length);0.1mm(thick)
- Female→8-10cm(length);0.2-0.3mm(thick)

Fig.1: Life cycle of *W. bancrofti*

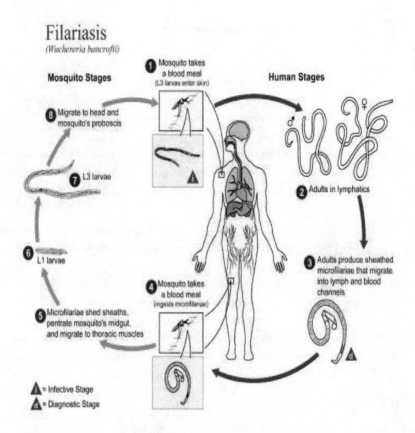

Fig.2: Microfilariae {male (short) and female (long)}.

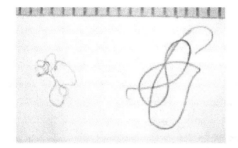

Fig.3: Microscopic examination of the blood smear

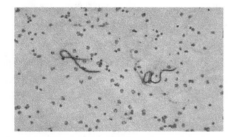

Fig: 4 Elephantiasis of leg

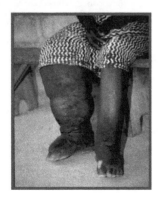

TRANSMISSION:

The most important species of vector is _Culex quinquefasciatus_. This mosquito, together with _Anopheles gambiae_ and _Anopheles funestus_, is the most important vector in sub-Saharan Africa. In Egypt, _Culex pipiens_ is the principal vector. _Culex_ mosquitoes lay their eggs in small groups on the water surface. _Mansonia_ mosquitoes (subgenus _Mansonioides_) are also vectors and are found in association with certain water plants. Transmission via mosquitoes means that there is very marked geographical heterogeneity.

After being sucked up by the mosquito, microfilaria reaches the abdominal stomach via the proboscis, pharynx and thoracic esophagus. Chitinous teeth in the foregut can mechanically damage aspirated microfilariae. These teeth are particularly pronounced in _Anopheles_ females. In the stomach, the parasites shed their sheath, penetrate the gastric wall and migrate via the haemocoel to the insect's thoracic muscles. After maturation, the immature worms migrate through the insect's head to the labium ("lower lip") of the proboscis. This stage is reached approximately 10 days after the blood meal. When the mosquito again sucks blood, the 1.2-1.6 mm long infective larvae break through the labella of the labium and then creep onto the skin (the labium is not inserted into the skin, in contrast to other mouthparts). If the parasite, now known as an infective larva, finds a portal of entry (e.g. the bite wound), it enters and is transported via the lymphatic. The insect's salivary glands play no direct role in transmission, in contrast to malaria.

Wuchereria bancrofti becomes adult in human lymphatic and lymph nodes. The worms are 0.2 mm wide and can be up to 10 cm long. They survive for up to 10 years. Approximately 6 to 12 months after infection, microfilariae appear in the circulation. Every day, the female produces numerous microfilariae (250 to 300 μm long and 8 μm wide). They are surrounded by an egg membrane (sheath). The membrane is sometimes very difficult to see in a microscopic preparation.

The minimum level of Mf which will permit infection of mosquitoes is not known. It is reported that a man with one Mf per 40 cu.mm of blood was infective to 2.6% of mosquitoes fed on him. On the other hand, when mosquitoes were fed on carriers having as many as 80 or more Mf per 20 cu.mm, the heavily infected mosquitoes did not survive when a number of MF began to reach maturity.

Filariasis is spread from infected persons to uninfected persons by mosquitoes. Adult worms live in an infected person's lymph vessels. The females release large numbers of very small worm larvae, which circulate in an infected person's bloodstream. When the person is

8

bitten by a mosquito, the mosquito can ingest the larvae. These develop in the mosquito and can then be spread to other people via mosquito bites. After a bite, the larvae pass through the skin, travel to the lymph vessels, and develop into adults, which live about 7 years. Then the cycle begins again[15].

FACTORS:

1. Host factors: **Man is the natural host.**

    a) AGE: - All ages are susceptible to infection. In endemic areas, filarial infection has been found even in infants aged less than 6 months. Infection rates rise within age up to 20-30 years and then the level falls off. After a few years with this plateau level, rates may decline in middle and old age. Filarial disease appears only in a small proportion in individuals over 10 years of age.

    b) SEX: - In most endemic areas, the Mf rate is higher in male than in females.

    c) MIGRATION: - The movement of people from place to place has led to the extension of filariasis into areas previously non-endemic.

    d) IMMUNITY: - Man may develop resistance to infection only after years of exposure.

2. Social Factors: Lymphatic filariasis is often associated with urbanization, industrialization, migration of people, illiteracy, poverty and poor sanitation.

3. Environmental Factors:

    i. CLIMATE: - It is an important factor in the epidemiology of filariasis. It influences the longevity and also determines the development of the parasite in the vector. The maximum prevalence of *Culex quinquefasciatus* was observed when the temperature was 28- 38 degree centigrade.

    ii. DRAINAGE: - The disease is associated with poor drainage.

    iii. TOWN PLANNING: - Inadequate sewage disposal and lack of town planning have aggravated the problem of Lymphatic filariasis.

    iv. The common breeding places of mosquitoes are soakage-pits, septic tanks, burrow pits, open ditches, cesspools.

4. AGENT FACTORS:

There are at least 8 species of filarial parasites that are specific to man. The following table summarizes them.

Table: 1.2 Agent factor

Organism	Vectors	Disease Produced
1. *Wuchereria bancrofti*	Culex mosqitoes	Lymphatic filariasis
2. *Brugia malayi*	Mansonia mosquitoes	Lymphatic filariasis
3. *Brugia timori*	Anopheles mosquitoes Mansonia mosqitoes	Lymphatic filariasis
4. *Onchocerca volvulus*	Simulum flies	Subcutaneous nodules; River blindness
5. *Loa loa*	Chryopses flies	Recurrent transient subcutaneous swellings
6. *T.perstans*	Culicoides	Probably rarely any clinical illness
7. *T. streptocerca*	Culicoides	Probably rarely any clinical illness
8. *Mansonella ozzardi*	Culicoides	Probably rarely any clinical illness

PROGRESSION OF LYMPHATIC FILARIASIS:

Prepatent Period

The prepatent period is known as the period between the entrance of the infective larva into the human host and the first appearance of microfilaria within the human host. Because detection of low levels of microfilariae can be so difficult, the prepatent period will vary depending on the duration of time spent in an endemic area, and the amount of exposure to the vector. Little is known about the prepatent period in humans, but tests done on primates show a period of 7-8 months for W. bancrofti and 2 months for B. malayi.

Incubation Period

The incubation period is known as the period between the entrance of the infective larva into the human host and the presentation of clinical symptoms or observable signs. This period of time is completely variable, and can be as short as 4 weeks or as long as 8-16 months.

Chronic Stage of Lymphatic Filariasis

The chronic stage of lymphatic filariasis patients is also completely variable. In some patients it develops quickly, while in others it does not. Some patients develop chronic symptoms while they have living microfilariae in their circulatory system while other patients develop chronic symptoms long after microfilariae and adult worms have died. The high variability associated with the development of chronic symptoms is a mystery to many, and research is currently exploring causal relationships between levels of microfilaria and chronic symptoms.

PATHOGENESIS

The adult worm induces an immunological reaction in humans. The basic lesion is a sterile inflammation around the worm, in and around the lymph nodes and lymph vessels. In the case of lymphangitis, there is often retrograde inflammation (centrifugal spread). This inflammation leads to obstruction of lymph vessels, resulting in temporary lymphostasis and lymphoedema. Following repeated attacks, irreversible damage to the lymphatic occurs with permanent "non-pitting" lymphoedema. Sometimes abscesses occur at the site of dead adult worms. There are also findings that indicate that adult worms can themselves directly attack the lymphatic (irrespective of the immunological response). Children born to microfilaraemic mothers have reduced immunological reactions to microfilaria antigens in comparison to children of non-infected mothers. This immunological tolerance lasts for many years after birth. Occasionally microfilariae penetrate the placenta, but this has no major consequences (microfilariae are not pathogenic). True congenital transmission does not occur. Microfilariae that are accidentally transmitted via a blood transfusion remain present in the recipient's blood for approximately one month. In humans with severe symptoms, low or no microfilaremia is found in most cases, whereas humans with high microfilaremia often have no symptoms. The reasons for this apparent paradox are that the pathology is caused by the patient's immunological response to the adult worms. If the reaction is violent, few adult worms and microfilariae survive, but considerable inflammation will occur with sequel. During infection with the filariae, the immunological response evolves. Down-regulation can occur and some patients do not produce any interferon-gamma after exposure to parasitic antigen. This is currently the subject of intense study.

The outcome of filarial infection varies in different persons. In some patients, especially from endemic areas, infection may be entirely asymptomatic, even with a high Mf count in their peripheral blood (20,000/ml). Such persons appear o tolerate Mf and do not mount an immune response against them, immune response being inhibited by immune suppressor cells.

In other persons particularly from non-endemic areas, infection may cause early clinical manifestations characterized by fever, lymphangitis and lymphadenitis with chills and recurrent febrile attack. They mount an immune response against the infection so Mf may not be demonstrable in them. The infective larvae that enter the human body through mosquito bite enter the lymphatic system where they molt and their body proteins, body secretions and other products, in some persons cause irritation directly or due to hypersensitivity and other immunological inflammation.

The typical manifestation of filariasis is caused by adult worms blocking the lymph nodes and vessels either mechanically or more commonly due to allergic inflammatory response to worm antigen secretions.

The affected lymph nodes are infiltrated with macrophages, eosinophils, lymphocytes and plasma cells and show endothelial hyperplasia. The vessel wall gets thickened and the lumen narrowed or occluded leading to lymph stasis and dilation of lymph vessels. The worms inside lymph nodes and vessels may cause granuloma formation with subsequent scarring and even calcification. Increased permeability of lymph vessels may lead to leakage of protein rich lymph into the tissues.

CLINICAL MANIFESTATIONS:

5 main categories of the filarial clinical spectrum have been recognized. These are:-

A. Asymptomatic microfilaremia.
B. Asymptomatic amicrofilaraemia.
C. Acute manifestations.
D. Allergic manifestations.
E. Chronic manifestations.

Among the more obvious symptoms, the acute, temporary signs and symptoms caused by inflammation should be distinguished from those resulting from chronic lymph tract obstruction.

A. Asymptomatic amicrofilaraemia:

In all endemic areas, a proportion of the population shows neither microfilaremia nor clinical manifestation of filarial infection and some of them have probably not been sufficiently exposed to the infective bites, whereas other persons may have been sufficiently exposed but do not have infection (as detectable by current diagnostic techniques); they may be immune or partially immune to infection. Still others in this group may have sub clinical infections (without microfilaremia), as indicated by the presence of filarial antigens in the blood.

B. Asymptomatic microfilaraemia:

Certain individuals in the population of an endemic area develop microfilaremia but without recognizable clinical manifestation of filariasis. Recent studies using lymphoscintigraphy have clearly shown that even in their asymptomatic state, these individuals have dilated lymphatic and compromised lymphatic functions.

C. Acute manifestations:

The acute clinical manifestations of lymphatic filariasis are characterized by periodic attacks of adenolymphangitis associated with fever and malaise. In males with bancroftian filariasis, this adenolymphangitis may be localized in the genitals and present as acute epididymo-orchitis. It is not certain whether some of these are episodes of adenolymphangitis triggered or accompanied by bacterial infection. Nevertheless, treatment with antibiotics reduces the frequency of such episodes and also prevents lymphoedema. Inflammatory nodules in the breast, scrotum or subcutaneous tissues (presumably reflecting inflammatory reactions around adult or developing worms) have also been reported as acute manifestation of infection. It includes constitutional symptoms like fever, chills, malaise and vomiting.

D. Allergic manifestations:

The metabolites of growing larvae ion highly reacting individuals may give rise to allergic manifestations like urticaria, fugitive swelling and lymphoedema.

Signs of **inflammation**:

1. Filarial fever 2. Adenolymphangitis (ADL) 3. Lymphadenitis.

1. Filarial Fever: Filarial lymphangitis is usually accompanied by a rise of temperature ranging from 103degree-104degree F which may continue for several days(3-5 days). The temperature comes down by crisis with profuse sweating. The fever is associated with a localized sign of inflammation of the lymphatic vessel where the adult worm lies. Examinations of blood show an increase of neutrophils, it may also reveal the presence of Mf, and transient leucocytosis. Irregular fever often occurs without external lymph node inflammation, as a result of inflammation of the deeper lymphatic and lymph nodes. The fever may recur irregularly for months or years after the patient leaves an endemic region.

2. Adenolymphangitis (ADL): Acute pain and inflammation in one or more lymph nodes (groin, axilla, elbow, neck). This is associated with fever and general malaise. Retrograde lymphangitis often occurs after 4 to 8 hours. There is centrifugal redness, pain and heat over the course of the lymph vessels. Pyogenic lymphangitis proceeds centripetal, not centrifugal. In most cases, the symptoms last 3-4 days. Each episode results in several days of incapacity for work. Acute lymphangitis is usually caused by allergic or inflammatory reaction to filarial infection, but may often be associated with streptococcal infection.

Causes of Lymphangitis:

1. Mechanical irritation- Movement of the adult parasite inside the lymphatic system.

2. Liberation of metabolites of the growing larvae in highly reacting individuals and secretion of some toxic fluid by fertilized females at the time of parturition.

3. Absorption of toxic products liberated from dead worms undergoing disintegration.

4. Bacterial infection Streptococci may appear as secondary invaders *(S.pyrogenes* and *S.aureus).*

Bacterial infection is mainly due to the accumulation of protein and the swelling and the decreased function of the lymph system, thus making it difficult for the body to fight germs and infections.

3. Lymphadenitis: Repeated episodes of acute lymphadenitis occur with fever very frequently. The inguinal nodes are most affected and auxiliary nodes less commonly. The swollen nodes may be painful and tender.

Causes of lymphatic obstruction:-

- Mechanical blocking of the lumen by dead worms (single or bunch) which act as embolus.

14

- Obliferative endolymphangitis Endothethial proliferation and inflammatory thickening of the walls of lymphatic vessels.
- Fibrosis of afferent lymph nodes draining a particular area.

Tropical pulmonary eosinophilia, Weingarten's syndrome:

Pulmonary symptoms are predominant: cough, dyspnoea, "asthmatic syndrome", blood eosinophil count is 3000-5000 cu mm. Chest X-rays very consistently show patchy infiltrates, in contrast to Loeffler's syndrome in which they are more fleeting. Sometimes the lymph nodes swell and spleenomegaly occurs. And there is marked eosinophilia. . Males are affected twice as often as females, and the disease is rarely seen in children. Extra pulmonary manifestations occur in about 15% of the patients, including mild to moderate splenomegaly, lymphadenopathy, and hepatomegaly. The syndrome is characterized by nocturnal paroxysmal cough, hypereosinophilia, elevated erythrocyte sedimentation rate, radiological evidence of diffuse miliary lesions or increased broncho-vascular markings, extremely high titer of filarial antibody (including1gE), and a good therapeutic response to DEC. Low grade fever and weight loss may be present.

In most cases lung function is impaired, with reduction in the vital capacity, total lung capacity, and residual volume. Hypereosinophilia is the most constant feature of this syndrome. Absolute eosinophilia counts generally range from 3000 to 50000 cells per mm^3 of blood, but the level of eosinophilia is not related to the severity of the syndrome. If untreated, tropical pulmonary eosinophilia progresses to a condition of chronic pulmonary fibrosis.TPE could be diagnosed by lung biopsy, test for filarial Ag which gives a strong positive result and patients respond promptly to DEC confirming the diagnosis.

Occult Filarisis:

The term "occult" or "cryptic" filarisis refers to filarial infection in which the clinical manifestations and Mf are not present. This term refers to the hypersensitivity reaction to Mf antigen and is characterized by massive eosinophilia and absence of Mf.

Adults produce Mf in lymph nodes, but they do not reach peripheral blood as they are destroyed in the tissues. In this unusual host reaction to filarial antigen, results in the formation of eosinophillic granulomas around a Mf or its remnants.Best example is TPE. Only a very small proportion of individuals in a community where filariasis is endemic develop occult forms of the

15

disease, condition in which the classical clinical manifestations are not present and where microfilariae are not found in the blood but may be found in the tissues.

Signs of **chronic obstruction**:

1. Hydrocoele.
2. Lymphoedema.
3. Chyluria.
4. Elephantiasis.
5. Lymphvarix.
6. Lymphorrhagia.

E. Chronic manifestations:

Hydrocele, lymphoedema, elephantiasis and chyluria are the main clinical pathological consequences of chronic bancroftian filariasis, the incidence and severity of these chronic manifestations increase with age. Chronic epididymitis, funiculitis (inflammatory swelling of the spermatic cord), and lymphoedematous thickening of the scrotal skin are also genital manifestations of chronic bancroftian filariasis.

Recurrent episodes of limb lymphoedema, first pitting oedema and then the chronic non-pitting oedema with loss of skin elasticity and fibrosis are the result of anatomical and/or functional blockage of the lymphatic. The legs are more commonly affected than the arms. Secondary infections of the skin (bacterial and fungal) are common, particularly in subjects who do not use foot wear.

1. Hydrocoele:

Hydrocoele often occurs in orchitis (inflammation of the testis). This is very common in an endemic region. Microfilariae are often found in hydrocoele fluid. Large hydrocoeles can be very inconvenient. Sexual incapacity associated with genital filariasis is a major concern for those infected. Shame, anxiety, sexual problems in marriage and social stigmatization are widespread. Note: lymph from the scrotum and the greater part of the penis drains towards the superficial inguinal lymph nodes that from the glands go principally to the deep inguinal nodes while from the testis it flows to the pre-aortic and retroperitoneal lumbar lymph nodes. The fluid is generally clear and straw coloured, but may sometimes be cloudy, milky or haemorrhagic.

2. Lymphoedema:

It follows successive attacks of lymphangitis and unusually starts swelling around the ankle, spreading to the back of foot and leg. It may also affect the arms, breast, scrotum, vulva or any other part of the body. Initially the oedema is pitting in nature, but in course of time, it becomes hard and non pitting.

It can be classified as follows:

a) Grade I lymphoedema: mostly pitting oedema; spontaneous reversible on elevation.

b) Grade II lymphoedema: mostly non-pitting oedema; not spontaneously reversible on elevation; skin normal

c) Grade III lymphoedema: mostly non-pitting oedema; not spontaneously reversible on elevation; skin thick.

d) Grade IV (elephantiasis): gross increase in volume in a grade II lymphoedema, with dermatosclerosis and papillomatous lesions.

3. Chyluria:

Chyluria is defined as the excretion of the chyle in the urinary tract. A minority of the affected subjects may also have gross haematuria. The basic pathophysiology is related to blockage of the retroperitoneal lymph nodes below the cisterna chyli with consequent reflux and flow of the intestinal lymph directly into the renal lymphatic, which may rupture and permit flow of chyle into the urinary tract. The resultant "milky urine" contains considerable quantities of lymph originating from the gastrointestinal tract. The condition is usually painless but large amounts of dietary lipids, proteins, and possibly fat soluble vitamins are excreted leading to weight loss. Microfilaraemia may or may not be present in these patients.

4. Elephantiasis:

This is delayed sequel to lymphangitis, obstruction and lymphoedema. Lymph exudates accumulating in the region stimulates connective tissue hypertrophy and hyperplasia. The part gets grossly enlarged and misshapen. The skin surface gets coarse with watery excretions. Cracks and fissures develop with secondary bacterial infection. Elephantiasis is mostly seen in legs, but may also involve arms, breast, scrotum, penis or vulva.

5. Lymphvarix: Dilation of lymph vessels commonly occur in the inguinal, scrotal, testicular and abdominal sites.

6. Lymphorrhagia:

Rupture of lymph vertices leads to the release of lymph or chyle. The clinical picture depends on the sites involved and includes lymph scrotum, chluria, and lymphocele.

Symptoms of other filariasis diseases:

- **Onchocerciasis** can cause pruritus, dermatitis, onchocercomata (subcutaneous nodules), and lymphadenopathies. The most serious manifestation consists of ocular lesions that can progress to blindness.
- **Loiasis** (*Loa loa*) is often asymptomatic. Episodic angioedema (Calabar swellings) and subconjunctival migration of an adult worm can occur.
- Infections by *Mansonella perstans*, while often asymptomatic, can be associated with angioedema, pruritus, fever, headaches, arthralgias, and neurologic manifestations.
- *Mansonella streptocerca* can cause skin manifestations including pruritus, papular eruptions and pigmentation changes. Eosinophilia is often prominent in filarial infections.
- *Mansonella ozzardi* can cause symptoms that include arthralgias, headaches, fever, pulmonary symptoms, adenopathy, hepatomegaly, and pruritus.

DIAGNOSIS:

1. Detection of Microfilaraemia:

Filariasis is usually diagnosed by identifying microfilariae on a Giemsa stained thick blood film. Blood must be drawn at night, since the microfilaria circulate at night (nocturnal periodicity), when their mosquito vector is most likely to bite. Also, decreased peripheral temperature, along with oxygen tension may attract more microfilariae.

Collecting blood from the individual for microscopic examination should be done during the night when the microfilariae are more numerous in the bloodstream. (Interestingly, this is when mosquitoes bite most frequently.) During the day microfilariae migrate to deeper blood vessels in the body, especially in the lung. If it is decided to perform the blood test during the day, the infected individual may be given a "provocative" dose of medication to provoke the microfilariae to enter the bloodstream. Blood then can be collected an hour later for examination.

DEC provocation test: Mf can be induced to appear in blood in the daytime by administrating diethylcarbamazine (DEC) 100gm orally. Mf begins to reach their peak within 15 minutes and begins to decrease 2 hours later. The blood may be examined one hour after administration.

Microscopic examination of the person's blood may reveal microfilariae. But many times, people who have been infected for a long time do not have microfilariae in their bloodstream. The absence of them, therefore, does not mean necessarily that the person is not infected. In these cases, examining the urine or hydrocele fluid or performing other clinical tests is necessary.

2. Demonstration of adult worms

Lymph node biopsies can be done to detect adult worms. Detecting the adult worms can be difficult because they are deep within the lymphatic system and difficult to get to. Biopsies usually are not performed because they usually don't reveal much information.

3. Immuno diagnosis:

Another method is the ICT filariasis card test (Immuno-Chromatographic Test). The test strip has monoclonal antibodies (AD12.1) at one end. When plasma containing parasite's antigens are added and the mixture allowed migrating towards the other end, antigen-antibody complexes will form. If the complexes are detected at the correct location, the test is positive.

A comparable test is the TropBio® test which detects circulating antigens by means of another monoclonal antibody (Og4C3). The technique is very simple (like ICT-test for malaria). There is no diurnal variation in the concentration of free circulating antigen so that nocturnal blood sampling is not necessary. It is a powerful test for studying the efficacy of chemotherapy. People who have no microfilariae in the blood but who do harbor live adult *W. bancrofti* test positive. People who recover no longer have circulating antigen in the blood.

4. Indirect test:

Blood count: - Hypereosinophilia is the most constant feature of this syndrome. Absolute eosinophilia counts generally range from 3000 to 50000 cells per mm^3 of blood, could detect TPE, a feature of inflammation of filariasis. (Eosinophil- 5-15%).

19

5. Xenodiagnosis:

Here, the mosquitoes are allowed to feed on the patient, and then their stomach dissected to demonstrate the Mf, two weeks late. Where other techniques may fail, this may succeed in detecting low density microfilaremia[16].

TREATMENT

(i)   DEC (Diethyl Carbamazine) is given in a dose of 6mg DEC/Kg body weight, for 12days for clearing microfilariae.

(ii)   Ivermectin (400 mcg/kg/d) is an equally potent microfilaricide, and the combination of DEC and ivermectin provides significant synergism.

(iii)   Albendazole (400mg/kg) acts predominantly on adult parasites leading to decreased micro filarial production.

(iv)   Currently, single dose Albendazole (400mg) and DEC (6mg/kg) is administered annually for 4-6 yrs, a regimen approved by WHO.

Prophylaxis

Good, enforced hygiene can dramatically reduce the number of complications. General cleanliness, washing with soap and disinfection of wounds are crucial. If bacterial super infection is present, this should be treated appropriately. There is often a fungal infection between the toes (athlete's foot), which acts as a portal of entry for various bacteria. Simple hygiene is important and should be stressed:

1.   Feet hygiene.

2.   Regular clipping of toe and finger nails.

3.   Regular application of Whitfield ointment.

4.   Prompt and appropriate attention to all injuries of the body.

5.   Chemical control of Mosquitoes.

6.   Removal of Pistia Plant.

7.   Minor Environmental measures.

Aim & Objectives

The objective of present study is to analyze the safety & acceptability of co-administration of high/low dose albendazole with DEC in microfilaraemic individuals by single dose oral administration & to assess the toxicological profile of standard dose and high dose regimen of Albendazole with DEC when administered by oral route to albino mice.

LITERATURE REVIEW

Lymphatic filariasis is caused by infection with one of three nematodes, *Wuchereria bancrofti, Brugia malayi, or Brugia timori.* These agents cause similar clinical syndromes. They are a major cause of disfigurement and disability in endemic areas, leading to significant economic and psychosocial impact.

In mainland India, *Wuchereria bancrofti* transmitted by the ubiquitous vector, *Culex quinquefasciatus,* has been the most predominant infection contributing to 99.4% of the problem in the country. The infection is prevalent in both urban and rural areas. *Brugia malayi* infection is mainly restricted to rural areas due to peculiar breeding habits of the vector associated with floating vegetation. *Mansonia (Mansonioides) annulifera* is the principal vector while *M (M) uniformis* is the secondary vector. The vectorial role of *M(M) Indiana* is very limited due to its low density. Both *W bancrofti* and *B malayi* infections in mainland India exhibit nocturnal periodicity of microfilaraemia. In 1974-75 diurnal subperiodic *W bancrofti* infection was discovered among aborigines, inhabiting Nicobar group of Andaman & Nicobar Islands. *Aedes (Finlaya) niveus* group of mosquitoes were incriminated as the vectors for this infection[9].

The clinical manifestations of LF may vary from one endemic area to another. Generally, the most common clinical form of the disease is hydrocele, with lymphoedema and elephantiasis occurs less commonly.In India and neighbouring countries, both hydrocele and lymphoedema are common. Other forms of the disease such as tropical pulmonary eosinophilia and chyluria occur less frequently. Hydrocele is not seen in areas affected by Brugian filariasis. The most significant discovery has been in the area of chronic disease, with understanding of the key role of bacterial infection in the occurrence of acute attacks and progression of the disease. It has become increasingly evident that good daily hygiene practices – such as washing the affected parts and simple exercises that increase lymph flow – may play an important part in progression of the early stages of lymphoedema, thus reducing acute attacks[10].

Until recently, diagnosis of filarial infection depended on the direct demonstration of the parasite (almost always microfilariae) in blood or skin specimens using relatively cumbersome techniques and having to take into account the periodicity (nocturnal or diurnal) of microfilariae in blood. Alternative methods based on detection of antibodies by immunodiagnostic tests did not prove satisfactory since they both failed to distinguish between active and past infections and had problems with specificity owing to their cross-reactivity with common gastrointestinal parasites and other organisms. Circulating filarial antigen (CFA) detection test is now regarded as the 'gold standard' for diagnosing *Wuchereria bancrofti* infections. The specificity of these assays is near complete, and the sensitivity is greater than that achievable by the earlier parasitedetection assays. Two commercial configurations of this assay are available, one based on enzyme-linked immunosorbent assay (ELISA) methodology that yields semi-quantitative results, and the other based on a simple immunochromatographic card test, yielding only qualitative (positive/negative) answers[11].

The estimates in 2001 indicate that about 473 million people are exposed to the risk of bancroftian infection and of these about 125 million live in urban areas and about 348 million in rural areas. About 31 million people are estimated to be harbouring microfilaria (mf) and over 23 million suffer from filaria disease manifestations. State of Bihar has highest endemicity (over 17%) followed by Kerala (15.7%) and Uttar Pradesh (14.6%). Andhra Pradesh and Tamil Nadu have about 10% endemicity. Goa showed the lowest endemicity (less than 1%) followed by Lakshadweep (1.8%), Madhya Pradesh (above 3%) and Assam (about 5%). The seven states namely Andhra Pradesh, Bihar, Kerala, Orissa, Uttar Pradesh, Tamil Nadu, and West Bengal, where MDA pilot trials are being undertaken, contribute over 86% of mf carriers and 97% of disease cases in the country[12].

Understanding the age and gender distribution of the disease is important to identify the target groups for intervention. The prevalence of infection and disease are significantly higher in males compared to females Young adults in age group of 15-44 recorded the highest prevalence of infection. This group also formed the predominant age class in the population.(Micheal et al.,1996) estimated that globally, this age class contributes to 58.5% of all microfilaria (mF) carriers, 47.2% of lymphoedema cases and 58.3% of hydrocele cases and constituted 46.9% of the total population. Children and young adults below the age of 20 years also record high prevalence infection, detected by newer techniques for antigenaemia. The prevalence in these individuals ranged between 6.74 in South India (VCRC unpublished data) and 7.70% in Ghana. This suggests that they are also infected, but do not exhibit mF in the night in peripheral blood for some or other reason. Therefore, coverage of mass treatment in these age classes will be crucial.

Prevalence of chronic disease increases monotonically from young adult age classes (about 15 years) onwards to reach a peak in older age classes due to a cumulative effect, as

23

chronically diseased persons remain lifelong diseased. The incidence of acute ADL also shows a similar age pattern as chronic disease prevalence, since episodes of ADL predominantly occur in people with severe chronic disease. Males record very high prevalence of disease particularly due to occurrence of hydrocele. However, if hydrocele is not considered, the patterns are similar for both genders. In stable endemic areas, the prevalence of chronic disease and hydrocele show an age dependent rise. A distinct monotonic increase in age prevalence is seen for hydrocele. In most Asian and African stable endemic sites, the prevalence of hydrocele can be as high as 50% in older age classes above 45 years of age. Meta-analyses in 1996 have also shown an age specific rise in hydrocele prevalence. However, as the total number of males in the age class of 15-44 is highest among all males in the endemic countries, this most productive age class accounts for 15.62 out of a total of 26.79 million hydrocele cases in the world. It is well known that ADL attacks form a part of the natural history of scrotal disease and that repeated acute attacks could lead to progression to the most severe forms, including lymph scrotum. These attacks are could be linked to the presence of superficial bacterial and fungal infections, as is the case also with lymphoedema of the legs; or due to parasite induced inflammation. Episodic attacks ADL (acute filarial disease) continue to occur in established cases of chronic disease and in fact are responsible for the progression of chronic disease[30].

Diethylcarbamazine (DEC) is an effective drug acting on the parasite (without report of resistance in past five decades) and mass annual single dose community drug administration with selective vector control could result in effective elimination of infection by interruption of transmission. This has led to the articulation of the World Health Assembly Resolution (1997) for global elimination of lymphatic filariasis. The WHO has now called for targeting 'filariasis elimination' by 2020 India is the largest LF endemic country and has targeted elimination by 2015Transmission control and disability/morbidity management/control are the two pillars of the global elimination strategy. For transmission control, mass annual single dose administration of DEC and or DEC + Albendazole to entire communities at risk of infection has been recommended. Recognizing that episodic acute adeno-lymphangitis (ADL) attacks are associated with the progression of lymphoedema through stages and these are caused by secondary bacterial infections, foot hygiene has been recommended as a morbidity management strategy for LF elimination.. However, morbidity management strategy needs to be evolved for LF patients who suffer from genito-urinary (GU) manifestations, the burden of which is larger compared to lymphoedema[31].

24

The International Task Force for disease eradication had identified lymphatic filariasis as one of the only seven infectious diseases considered eradicable or potentially eradicable. The single dose mass therapy with DEC has been found to be as effective as 12 day therapy, as a public health measure, with lesser side effects thus enhancing public compliance, decreased delivery costs. It does not require complex management and infrastructure. It can be integrated into the existing primary health care system for delivery compliance. Single dose mass administration annually in combination with other techniques has already eliminated lymphatic filariasis from Japan, Taiwan, South Korea and Solomon Islands and markedly reduced the transmission in China[13].

CLINICAL PHARMACOLOGY (ALBENDAZOLE)

Pharmacokinetics

Absorption:

Albendazole is poorly absorbed from the gastrointestinal tract due to its low aqueous solubility. Albendazole concentrations are negligible or undetectable in plasma as it is rapidly converted to the sulfoxide metabolite prior to reaching the systemic circulation. The systemic anthelmintic activity has been attributed to the primary metabolite, albendazole sulfoxide. Oral bioavailability appears to be enhanced when albendazole is coadministered with a fatty meal.

Distribution:

Albendazole sulfoxide is 70% bound to plasma protein and is widely distributed throughout the body; it has been detected in urine, bile, liver and cerebral spinal fluid (CSF). Concentrations in plasma were 3- to 10-fold and 2- to 4-fold higher than those simultaneously determined in cyst fluid and CSF, respectively.

Metabolism and Excretion:

Albendazole is rapidly converted in the liver to the primary metabolite, albendazole sulfoxide, which is further metabolized to albendazole sulfone and other primary oxidative metabolites that have been identified in human urine. Following oral administration, albendazole has not been detected in human urine. Urinary excretion of albendazole sulfoxide is a minor elimination pathway with less than 1% of the dose recovered in the urine. Biliary elimination presumably accounts for a portion of the elimination as evidenced by biliary concentrations of albendazole sulfoxide similar to those achieved in plasma.

25

Microbiology:

The principal mode of action for albendazole is by its inhibitory effect on tubulin polymerization which results in the loss of cytoplasmic microtubules.

In the specified treatment indications albendazole appears to be active against the larval forms of the some organisms.

PATIENT INFORMATION

Patients should be advised that:

- Albendazole may cause fetal harm, therefore, women of childbearing age should begin treatment after a negative pregnancy test.
- Women of childbearing age should be cautioned against becoming pregnant while on albendazole or within 1 month of completing treatment.
- During albendazole therapy, because of the possibility of harm to the liver or bone marrow, routine (every 2 weeks) monitoring of blood counts and liver function tests should take place.
- Albendazole should be taken with food.

SIDE EFFECTS: Nausea, vomiting, abdominal pain, headache, or temporary hair loss may occur.

PRECAUTIONS:

- Before taking albendazole, tell your doctor or pharmacist if you are allergic to it; or to other benzimidazole anthelmintic drugs (e.g., mebendazole); or if you have any other allergies.
- Before using this medication, tell your doctor or pharmacist your medical history, especially of: liver disease, biliary tract problems (e.g., blockage), blood/bone marrow disorders.
- This medication may cause liver problems. Because drinking alcohol increases the risk of liver problems, limit alcoholic beverages while using this medication. Check with your doctor or pharmacist for more information.
- During pregnancy, this medication should be used only when clearly needed. It may harm an unborn baby. Women of child-bearing age should have a negative pregnancy test before starting this medication. It is not known if this medication passes into breast milk. Consult your doctor before breast-feeding.

26

CLINICAL PHARMACOLOGY (DEC)

Diethylcarbamazine (DEC) is a first-line agent for control and treatment of lymphatic filariasis and for therapy of tropical pulmonary eosinophilia (TPE) caused by *Wuchereria bancrofti* and *Brugia malayi*. Although this agent is partially effective against onchocerciasis and loiasis, it can cause serious reactions to affected microfilariae in both infections. For this reason, ivermectin has replaced diethylcarbamazine for therapy of onchocerciasis. Despite its toxicity, diethylcarbamazine remains the best drug available to treat loiasis. Annual single doses of both diethylcarbamazine and albendazole show considerable promise for the control of lymphatic filariasis in geographic regions where onchocerciasis and loiasis are not endemic.

Chemistry:

Diethylcarbamazine (HETRAZAN) is formulated as the water-soluble citrate salt containing 51% by weight of the active base. Because the compound is tasteless, odorless, and stable to heat, it also can be taken in the form of fortified table salt containing 0.2% to 0.4% by weight of the base.

Anthelmintic Action:

Microfilarial forms of susceptible filarial species are most affected by diethylcarbamazine, which elicits rapid disappearance of these developmental forms of *W. bancrofti, B. malayi,* and *L. loa* from human blood. The drug causes microfilariae of *O. volvulus* to disappear from skin but does not kill microfilariae in nodules that contain the adult (female) worms. It does not affect the microfilariae of *W. bancrofti* in a hydrocele, despite penetration into the fluid. The mechanism of action of diethylcarbamazine on susceptible microfilariae is not well understood, but the drug appears to exert a direct effect on *W. bancrofti* microfilariae by causing organelle damage and apoptosis .There is evidence that diethylcarbamazine kills worms of adult *L. loa* and probably adult *W. bancrofti* and *B. malayi* as well. However, it has little action against adult *O. volvulus*. The mechanism of filaricidal action of diethylcarbamazine against adult worms is unknown. Some studies suggest that diethylcarbamazine compromises intracellular processing and transport of certain macromolecules to the plasma membrane .The drug also may affect specific immune and inflammatory responses of the host by undefined mechanisms .

27

Absorption, Fate, and Excretion:

Diethylcarbamazine is absorbed rapidly from the gastrointestinal tract. Peak plasma levels occur within 1 to 2 hours after a single oral dose, and the plasma half-life varies from 2 to 10 hours, depending on the urinary pH. Metabolism is both rapid and extensive.A major metabolite, diethylcarbamazine-*N*-oxide, is bioactive. Diethylcarbamazine is excreted by both urinary and extraurinary routes; more than 50% of an oral dose appears in acidic urine as the unchanged drug, but this value is decreased when the urine is alkaline. Indeed, alkalinizing the urine can elevate plasma levels, prolong the plasma half-life, and increase both the therapeutic effect and toxicity of diethylcarbamazine .Therefore; dosage reduction may be required for people with renal dysfunction or sustained alkaline urine.

Therapeutic Uses:

Dosages of diethylcarbamazine citrate used to prevent or treat filarial infections have evolved empirically and vary according to local experience. Recommended regimens differ according to whether the drug is used for population-based chemotherapy, control of filarial disease, or prophylaxis against infection.

W. bancrofti, B. malayi, and B. timori. The standard regimen for the treatment of LF traditionally has been a 12-day, 72-mg/kg (6 mg/kg per day) course of diethylcarbamazine. In the United States, it is common practice to administer small test doses of 50 to 100 mg (1 to 2 mg/kg for children) over a 3-day period prior to beginning the 12-day regimen. However, a single dose of 6 mg/kg had comparable macrofilaricidal and microfilaricidal efficacy to the standard regimen. Single-dose therapy may be repeated every 6 to 12 months, as necessary.

For mass treatment with the objective of reducing microfilaremia to subinfective levels for mosquitoes, the introduction of diethylcarbamazine into table salt (0.2% to 0.4% by weight of the base) has markedly reduced the prevalence, severity, and transmission of lymphatic filariasis in many endemic areas. A major advance was the discovery that diethylcarbamazine given annually as a single oral dose of 6 mg/kg was most effective in reducing microfilaremia when coadministered with either albendazole (400 mg) or ivermectin (0.2 to 0.4 mg/kg) .Adverse reactions to microfilarial destruction, greater after the oral diethylcarbamazine tablet than the table salt preparation, usually are well tolerated. However, mass chemotherapy with diethylcarbamazine should *not* be used in regions where onchocerciasis or loiasis coexist because, even in the table salt formulation, the drug may induce severe reactions related to parasite burden in these infections.

28

Toxicity and Side Effects:

Below a daily dose of 8 to 10 mg/kg, direct toxic reactions to diethylcarbamazine are rarely severe and usually disappear within a few days despite continuation of therapy. These reactions include anorexia, nausea, headache, and at high doses, vomiting. Major adverse effects result directly or indirectly from the host response to destruction of parasites, primarily microfilariae.

Precautions and Contraindications:

Population-based chemotherapy with diethylcarbamazine should be avoided in areas where onchocerciasis or loiasis is endemic, although the drug can be used to protect foreign travelers from these infections. Pretreatment with glucocorticoids and antihistamines often is undertaken to minimize indirect reactions to diethylcarbamazine that result from dying microfilariae. Dosage reduction must be considered for patients with impaired renal function or persistent alkaline urine[17].

Study in Microfilaraemic Individuals

STUDY DESIGN AND METHODS

RMRC, Bhubaneswar:

The study was carried out as an additional observation of the ongoing activity of RMRC, Bhubaneswar; Orissa. It is a Constituent Organization of Indian Council of Medical Research (ICMR) working in the field of clinico-epidemiological & immunological profiles of lymphatic filariasis for last 25 years. Besides research in other areas the centre has undertaken several clinical trials under WHO.

The center has already established several field areas nearby, where filariasis is endemic suitable for both long term & short term studies. RMRC runs an out-patients clinic at Capital Hospital, Bhubaneswar with facilities for lab diagnosis & treatment including morbidity management facility. This centre has linkages with the Medical Colleges of the state in relation to the patient database, OPD & in-patient facility & scientific interactions in relevant projects.

Study area site:

For selection of subjects for the clinical trial, villages around Bhatimunda under Tangi PHC of Cuttack district of Orissa (endemic for filariasis) had been identified.

Subjects enrollment:

Subjects were taken into the study those who fulfilled certain inclusion criteria (CRF-1 of Appendix-II) which are described as follows:

1. age between 18yrs to 55yrs from both the genders
2. not pregnant or breastfeeding by history
3. willing to spend 3 days in wards of the hospitals at each site
4. willing to undergo night time blood draws every 6 months for 2 yrs
5. having ability to understand and sign the **informed consent**
6. also having Hb levels >9 g/dl, Cr <1.2 mg/dl, ALT < 30 U/L
7. and not having any history of allergy towards albendazole and DEC

The screening consent form (Appendix-I) explained orally by the study investigator. Volunteers signed the consent to indicate their willingness to participate in the screening procedure. Based on the results of night time microfilarial counts, volunteers with microfilarial counts greater than 50mf/ml of blood identified & informed consent was obtained.

A brief clinical examination & medical history (CRF-3 of Appendix-II) of the volunteers were recorded. Intravenous blood samples (2-3ml) were collected aseptically from

30

individuals between 9pm and 2am for blood microfilarial counts, circulating filarial antigen in the blood, eosinophil count, hemoglobin level, serum creatinine, ALT (CRF- 4 of Appendix-II).

Eligible volunteers recruited for the analysis of safety & acceptability of co-administration of different dosage combinations were divided into different arms (open randomized clinical trial) which involves comparison of efficacy of standard dose of albendazole (400mg) with DEC (300mg) versus high dose of albendazole (800mg) with DEC (300mg).

Treatment groups and dosing schedule:

After the baseline screening examinations those subjects had microfilaria count **greater than 50 mf/ml of blood** were identified and admitted to KIMS Hospital, BBSR. Drug allocation was done as per the treatment arm pre defined for each subject-Id & they were divided randomly into the following groups:

> **Standard dose group:** This group of subjects was taken 400 mg of albendazole and DEC (300 mg).

> **Double-dose group:** This group of subjects was taken 800 mg of albendazole and DEC (300 mg).

The Global Program for the Elimination of Lymphatic Filariasis (the non-profit agency that provides these drugs for the mass treatment program) provided study drugs.

Preparation of Mf slides:

Laboratory confirmation of diagnosis is necessary to identify asymptomatic patients and those with non-symptomatic patients. The time during which the night blood is to be collected is between 8:30 pm – 12 midnight.

Clearing of microscopic slides: (New and used)

New slides:

Clean new slides with tissue paper or muslin cloth to remove dust.

Used slides:

• 30 ml liquid soap or 75g of powdered soap added to 3-4 liters of water is sufficient to clean approximately 400 slides.

- Used slides were soaked in the above solution for 12-24 hours.
- The slides were rinsed thoroughly with distilled water.
- The slides were dried and wiped with a clean piece of muslin cloth.
- 25 slides/packet were wrapped in brown paper and stored in a clean dry place.

Preparation of a blood smear:

The blood smear is made from 20µl (4-5 drops) of blood by finger prick. The smear is made at night between 8:30pm – midnight.

Equipment Required:

- Clean glass slides
- Disposable lancets
- Cotton wool
- Clean cloth or handkerchief
- Slide box for 25 or 50 slides
- Spirit or anti-septic solution
- Markers
- Ball point pen
- Packing paper and rubber band

METHOD:

First Step:

1. The ring finger/third finger of the hand of the patient.
2. The fingertip was wiped with a cotton wool dipped in spirit.
3. With the palm held upwards, and pressure applied gently, drops of blood were taken onto a slide.
4. The fingertip was again wiped with a cotton wool dipped in spirit.
5. The fingertip is then allowed to dry.

Second Step:

1. Another slide was taken with smooth edges and was used as a spreader.
2. Using the edges of the spreader, a thick film (20mm wide and 30mm long) was made.
3. The slide was marked using a marker.
4. The slide was allowed to dry flat.

Third Step: The dried slide was placed in a clean slide box or wrapped in a clean paper.

Fourth Step: On the following day, the same slide number (I.D. number) was re-written with a marker in the middle of the thick smear before dehaemoglobinization.

Staining and Examination of Blood Smears:

Blood smears should be dehaemoglobinized and stained preferably within 12 hours. The smears prepared in the preceding night should be stained during the next day and not later than 48 hours.

METHOD:-

Step 1: DEHAEMOGLOBINIZATION:

1. Dried smears were immersed in a beaker containing water for 2-5 minutes.
2. The smear was rinsed again with clean water.
3. The smears were allowed to dry.

Step 2: FIXING:

1. The smear was dipped completely in jar/beaker containing 2% acid alcohol (2 parts of conc. HCl and 98 parts of methanol by volume) for a second.
2. The smear was air-dried.

Step 3: STAINING:

1. The slide was dipped in a beaker containing JSB-1 stain for 40-60 seconds.
2. The smear was washed with buffer water in beaker and the slide was allowed to air dry.

Microscopic examination of the blood smear:

The stained slide was placed on the microscope's stage with the smear upwards and smear was viewed under 10X objective.

Plan for monitoring subjects:

Baseline medical history, vital signs checked just prior to administration of study drugs i.e. albendazole & DEC. If the vital signs are abnormal, the person was not allowed to move from the screening to the randomization part of study (CRF-5&6 of Appendix-II). Pregnancy testing performed in women of childbearing age (rapid urine pregnancy test) prior to drug administration. Women found to be pregnant during course of study didn't receive any further doses of albendazole & DEC (CRF- 7 of Appendix-II). Vital sign monitoring-6 hourly, recording of reported AEs, Management of AEs done to follow up of the study subjects (48 hours) at hospital. Follow up subjects supervised at village level in third and seventh day (In between when necessary).

The enrolled patient with hydroceles/lymph node enlargement was subjected to ultrasound examination for adult worm nests which evaluated as an additional documentary feature for efficacy of the drug on the adult. In those subjects with detectable worm nests ("filarial dance signs"), ultrasound repeated within 3days following treatment (CRF- 8 of Appendix-II).

The following questions were put to subjects related to their awareness, willingness, knowledge about filariasis, past history etc before administration of drug.

Sample questionnaire form before drug administration:

Subject I.D No: Age: Sex: Wt:
Questionnaire
1) Do you think that your participation to this programme will be beneficial to you?   2) Do you know the main causes of filariasis?   3) Do you aware of filariasis?   4) Do you know the filariasis control programme?   5) Did you have taken albendazole or DEC within the past 6 months?   6) Do you have any history of benzimidazole allergy?   7) Do you have any history of DEC allergy?   8) Are you an alcoholic?   9) Are you pregnant/ breast feeding women?   10) Do you suffer from any other disease?

Drug administration and follow up:

Study drugs i.e. DEC, Albendazole tablets, from GSK Pharmaceutical Ltd. administered orally to subjects after breakfast between 8:30 a.m. to 9:00 a.m. (CRF-11 of Appendix-II). Also some data related to dosage form, regimen, side effects in the form of questionnaire were put to the study subjects after administration of drugs.

Sample questionnaire form after drug administration:

Subject I.D No: Age: Sex: Wt:
Questionnaire

1) Do you know about the signs & symptoms of filariasis?
 2) Are you a regular user of net/ mosquito coil?
 3) Do you think filariasis can be cured?
 4) Do you know the name of drugs used for treatment of filariasis?
 5) Did you have any difficulties during swallowing the tablets?
 6) Would you like to prefer chewable tablets?
 7) What would you like?
       • Either taking the two medicines in two divided doses
       • Or once in a day
 8) Would you like to take DEC 100mg three times a day?
 9) During the past year, how many times you have visited a doctor/been administered to a hospital?
 10) Did you suffer from any side effects after taking tablets?

Reporting of Adverse Events:

An adverse event (AE) is any undesirable experience / unwanted effect that occur in a patient or to a study subject during the course of clinical trial with the use of a medicine / investigational product. An adverse event is determined to be "serious" based on study subject/ event outcome usually associated with experience that pose a threat to a patient/ subjects life or functioning. All data entered into the case report form (CRFs) which are the source document (CRF-15of Appendix-II).

Toxicity management:

Most adverse effects of treating LF with these drugs were associated with systemic and local reactions to dying parasites. Side effects such as fever, headache, coughing, and a lightheaded feeling were fairly common in LF patients and last 1-3 days. Postural hypotension and nausea/vomiting were less common. These symptoms were self limited and can be treated with rest and oral acetaminophen. A minority of patients had been reported to develop nodules along lymphatic vessels and lymph nodes. Treatment with diethylcarbamazine occasionally resulted in reversible lymphedema. This had not been reported with the combination of Albendazole/DEC to date.

Local side effects are believed to be caused by host reactions to dying filarial worms. Even though these were expected toxicities, all non-serious adverse events was recorded on the case report forms (CRF-16 of Appendix-II) and reported to the Institutional Review Board (IRB) at the time of annual review.

Post treatment follow-up of the study subjects:

At the conclusion of the study (following administration of the final dose of Albendazole& DEC in the study) , all subjects treated with standard dose of Albendazole &DEC in collaboration with the Indian National Programme for the Elimination of Lymphatic Filariasis, that provides yearly DEC& Albendazole. The individuals receiving the treatment regimens in the in-patient facility at hospital (3 days hospitalization) followed regularly at their villages throughout the study period. On ethical grounds they also provided clinical advice and treatment for other minor illnesses if encountered during the study period by the physician of the research team.

Microfilariae levels as well as measures of adult worm burden will be studied in a periodic fashion every six months for two years to determine whether higher dose or more frequent regimen is more effective.

RESULTS

The safety & acceptability of co-administration of high/low dose of albendazole with DEC in microfilaraemic individuals were observed & analyzed.

A. Screening for microfilarimia

- Number of villages screened   –   7
- Total population screened (18-55 years) -   1011
- Number of microfilarimics identified –   92

B. Screening for eligibility and enrollment

- Number screened   –   51
- Number satisfying inclusion criteria –   51(39 male & 12 female)
- Drug allocation done -   51(33 standard & 18 high
                                      dose group)
- Number of subjects recorded for AE-   51

A total number of 92 individuals (aged 18-55yrs) with microfilarimics were identified from a total population of 1011. Of which 51 Subjects were satisfying inclusion criteria in this study; 51 subjects were screened; data were collected & recorded from 7 villages. Among them; 39 subjects were found to be males & rest were females. Drugs were given to a population of 51.

TABLE: 4.1 Baseline Parameters of enrolled subjects

Parameters	Value (mean)
Age in years	18-45(28.9)
Sex	Male- 39; Female – 12
MF count/ml	54 -3000 +
Serum Creatinine(mg/dl)	0.4 -1.2 (0.4)
Serum ALT(u/l)	13.6 – 29.8 (13.65)
Hemoglobin (gm %)	10.2 – 16.9 (10.6)
Eosinophil (%)	2 – 16 (10)
USG + ve for FDS	31/51(62%)

Prior to the administration of Albendazole & DEC a brief clinical examination & medical history was recorded for volunteers. Intravenous blood samples (2-3ml) collected aseptically from the individuals for microfilarial count, serum creatinine, serum ALT, haemoglobin, eosinophil. Then their mean values were calculated.

The enrolled patients with hydroceles / lymphnode enlargement were subjected to ultrasound examination for adult worm nest. 31 subjects were found to be positive for filarial dance sign from 51 subjects.

Drug administration and follow up:

Study drugs i.e. DEC (300mg) & Albendazole (400mg & 800mg) tablets, from GSK Pharmaceutical Ltd. administered orally to the respective groups of subjects after breakfast between 8:30 a.m. to 9:00 a.m.

TABLE: 4. 2   Post drug evaluation:

Parameters	DEC 300 mg+ ALB 400mg (n=33)	DEC 300mg + ALB 800mg (n= 18)
No. of subjects with Adverse events	23 (69 %)	11 (62 %)
No. of subjects with SAE	0	0
Absence of FDS in 3rd day (out of baseline FDS positives)	6/22(27.27%)	5/9(55.56%)
MF clearance*at 6th month	3/9(33.33%)	4/5(80%)

* Data from 14 subjects completing six month follow up

An adverse event (AE) can be categorized into as serious or non serious. After the administration of drugs subjects were observed & recorded from all the subjects for adverse events like fever, head reeling, headache, fatigue, testicular inflammation, and subcutaneous nodule, dizziness. 33 subjects were under the category of standard dose & rest was under double dose group from total population. The numbers of subjects with AEs in standard group were 23 out of total population of 33 & in double dose group were 11 out of 18 populations. It was seen that there was no serious adverse event (SAE) like death, life threatening event observed during the study in either of the group. Filarial dance sign (FDS) absent in 3rd day of monitoring the subjects was 6 out of 22 population of standard drug group & 5 from 9 subjects of double dose group (out of 31 baseline FDS positives).

MF clearance was found to be 3 out of 9 in standard group & 4 out of 5 in other group from a total of 14 subjects at 6th month follow up.

TABLE: 4.3 Adverse Events (n=34):

Parameters	Frequency (%)	Mean Duration of onset	Mean Duration of persistence
Fever	12(35.3)	10 hrs	11 hrs
Head reeling	4(11.7)	8 hrs	14 hrs
Headache	7(20.5)	9 hrs	14 hrs
Fatigue	2(6)	6 hrs	26 hrs
Testicular inflammation	10(29.4)	96 hrs	140 hrs

Parameters	Frequency (%)	Mean Duration of onset	Mean Duration of persistence
Subcutaneous nodule	1(2.9)	98 hrs	150 hrs
Dizziness	3(8.82)	6 hrs	22 hrs

* All received symptomatic treatment and recovered.

Different parameters like fever, head reeling, headache, fatigue, testicular inflammation, and subcutaneous nodule, dizziness were observed & frequency of them was recorded. These symptoms were self limited and can be treated with rest and oral acetaminophen. All received symptomatic treatment and recovered well.

TABLE: 4.4   Mf Count at baseline and 6months after drug in subjects followed

SL. NO.	Treatment Arm	Mf. Count	
		Pre drug	Post drug (6month)
1.	S	273	648
2.	S	228	00
3.	S	56	00
4.	S	568	405
5.	S	364	31
6.	S	41	00
7.	S	391	245
8.	S	646	392
9.	S	293	180
10.	H	445	00
11.	H	560	00
12.	H	347	00
13.	H	201	00
14.	H	972	258

*S= Standard Group, H= High Dose Group

The above table describes about mf Count at baseline and 6months after drug in subjects followed from the two treatment arms. MF clearance means total clearance in mf count in blood. MF clearance was found to be 3 out of 9(i.e. 33.33%) in standard group & 4 out of 5 (i.e. 80%) in other group from a total of 14 subjects at 6th month follow up.

Study in albino mice

STUDY DESIGN AND METHODS

Toxicity Study:

It is a study in which a single dose of the drug is used in each animal on one occasion only for the determination of gross behavior. The substances are administered orally to a group of experimental animals at one of the defined doses.

Requirements:

Animals:

After necessary approval (06/10/IAEC) from Institutional animal ethics committee (IAEC) of Royal college of Pharmacy and Health Sciences, Berhampur, the work was undertaken during April-2010 to May-2010.

Twelve numbers of albino mice (6 males & 6 females) were brought from the animal house of the Royal college of Pharmacy and Health Sciences, Berhampur. Male & female animals were kept separately in Polypropylene cages with paddy as the bedding at room temperature with relative humidity 30-70% in 12 hours light and 12 hours dark period. They fed pellet diet & aquaguard pure water in feeding bottle *ad libitum*. Also they were acclimated in laboratory seven days prior to initiation of the treatment. The animals were selected randomly & divided into 3 groups such that each group contains 2 male & 2 female albino mice. They were found healthy during check up. Individual animal body weight was ±20% of group mean body weight and group mean body weights of all the groups was approximately equal. Animals were identified by cage number and individual marking on fur.

> ➤ **Justification for selection of Albino mice for the Study:**

1) One of the rodent species recommended as test system for the use in toxicity studies,
2) Widely used throughout industry for the evaluation of toxicity of various products.

> ➤ **Route of Administration:** p.o, once on day 1.

> ➤ **Reason for Choice of oral route:**

1) The dosage can be accurately administered,
2) One of the proposed routes for toxicity testing.

Chemicals:

Albendazole 400 mg, DEC 100mg from GSK Pharmaceutical Ltd. were purchased from local market for the study.

Instruments:

Semi autoanalyzer-3000Evolution (Tulip), Haemometer (MARIENFELD, GERMANY), Microscope.

Extrapolation of mice dose from human dose[53]:

Conversion of dose for any animal from other is as per the surface area. Small animals have a big surface relative to weight from which heat is lost. To maintain body temperature relatively more heat must be produced. Hence the metabolic rate is more in mouse (180kcal/kg), than in rat (90), dog (36), and man (27). The dose to be given to a particular species on the basis of surface area can be extrapolated by referring to table 30.2 from Toxicity studies in *Fundamentals of Experimental Pharmacology* by M. N. Ghosh. To determine absolute dose for a species in column, absolute dose given to a species in a row is multiplied by factor given at intersection of relevant row & column. Thus an effect is produced in a 12 kg dog by a dose of 10 mg/kg; the absolute dose to the dog is 120 mg. Extrapolated to man by surface area, the effect might be expected at a dose of 120 mg × 3.1 = 372 mg, as opposed to 700 mg, given by the ratio of weights.

- For absolute dose **400mg/kg of Albendazole** in man; Extrapolated to mice at a dose of: 400mg × 0.0026 = 1.04 mg/20gm (**52mg/kg**).
- For absolute dose **800mg/kg of Albendazole** in man; Extrapolated to mice at a dose of: 800mg × 0.0026 = 2.08mg/20gm (**104mg/kg**)
- For absolute dose **300mg/kg of DEC** in man; Extrapolated to mice at a dose of: 300mg × 0.0026 = 0.78mg/20gm (**39mg/kg**).

Individual doses were calculated based on their body weights & doses were administered accordingly.

Vehicle: Distilled water (10ml/kg)

Dose volume: Maximum upto 10ml/kg

Administration: The drugs were administered once, orally by oral feeding needle to mice that have been fasted for 18 h. After the administration, food may be with held for a further 2 hours in mice.

Drug treatment protocol:

All the animals were divided into 3 groups (n=4). They were administered the drugs as per following schedule:

Table: 5.1 Drug treatment protocol

Sl. No.	Group	Drug/Dose	Dose levels (mg/kg)	No. of mice	
				Male	Female
I	Control	Distilled Water	10ml/kg	2	2
II	Standard	Albendazole +DEC	52+39	2	2
III	High dose	Albendazole +DEC	104+39	2	2

*DEC=300mg, Albendazole=400mg&800mg as human dose.

TOXICITY STUDY:

METHOD:

After oral administrations of different drugs to respective groups, the animals were observed continuously for 2 hours and then occasionally for further 4 hours and finally overnight mortality recorded. Behavior of the animals and any other toxic symptoms also observed for 72 h. and the animals were kept under observation upto 14 days.

OBSERVATIONS:

The following observations were recorded during the study period.

1. Mortality:

All animals were observed continuously for 2 hours and then occasionally for further 4 hours and finally overnight mortality recorded. All the animals were kept under observation upto

14 days and observed twice a day during the period of study. Moribund animals sacrificed and necropsy was carried out.

2. Clinical Signs:

A careful cage side examination made at least once each day. Provisional additional observations were made daily with appropriate actions taken to minimize loss of animals to the study, e.g. necropsy or refrigeration of those animals found dead, and isolation or sacrifice of weak or moribund animals, to ensure that not more than 10% of the animals in any study group lost from the test due to cannibalism, autolysis of tissues, misplacement, and similar management problems.

Clinical signs of toxicity recorded as they were observed including the time of onset, degree and duration. Cage side observations were including, but not be limited to, changes in: Skin and fur, Eyes and mucous membranes, respiratory systems, circulatory system, autonomic and central nervous system, Somatomotor activity and behaviour pattern.

3. Body Weight:

All the animals weighed initially before administration of drugs and on 7th day and 14th day. In addition, weights were recorded at the time of necropsy.

4. Food Intake:

The food intakes of the animals were measured before and after the drug treatment on weekly basis. Food consumed by animals per cage recorded and the food consumed by each animal calculated.

5. Clinical Laboratory Investigations:

At termination of study i.e. on 15th day, blood samples were withdrawn, from orbital sinus of all the animals, fasted overnight. The following haematological and biochemical investigations carried out.

a) Haematology: The haematological study included the following parameters

> Hb   : Hemoglobin

Differential count shall be done manually by using Leishmann's Staining method

> N   : Neutrophils
> L   : Lymphocytes
> E   : Eosinophils
> M   : Monocytes
> B   : Basophils

b) Clinical Biochemistry:

Semi autoanalyser 3000Evolution (Tulip) was used to determine the values of the following parameters.

➤ Glucose, SGOT, SGPT, Creatinine, Serum cholesterol, HDL, LDL, Triglyceride & VLDL.

6. Pathology:

Necropsy & Organ Weights: All the animals surviving at the end of treatment were sacrificed and examined for gross lesions. All animals which succumb during the course of treatment were examined for gross lesions. Different organs i.e. liver, kidney, spleen, and heart from all animals were dissected free of fat and weighed.

STATISTCS:

The statistical methods used to analyze the following data:

  a)   Body weight,

  b)   Food consumption,

  c)   Organ weights and

  d)   Clinical laboratory data.

All data's were expressed MEAN±SEM and student's t-test was applied for comparing the level of significant ($p < 0.05$) between the groups.

RESULTS

Acute toxicity study was carried out by taking 12 numbers of mice & divided into 3 groups; each containing 2 males & 2 females. During the toxicity study all groups were found to be active & healthy. Observations were found as following:

1. Mortality:

All animals were observed continuously for 2 hours and then occasionally for further 4 hours and finally overnight mortality recorded. No mortality was found during the oral toxicity study in mice.

3. Signs of Acute Toxicity:

TABLE: 5.2: Signs of acute toxicity

Signs Of Acute Toxicity	Group-I	Group-II	Group-III
1. Tremor	- - - -	- - - -	- - - -
2. Clonic convulsion	- - - -	- - - -	- - - -

45

Signs Of Acute Toxicity	Group-I	Group-II	Group-III
3. Tonic extension	- - - -	- - - -	- - - -
4. Straub reaction	- - - -	+ - - -	- + - -
5. Muscle spasm	- - - -	- - - -	- - - -
6. Catatonia	- - - -	- - - -	- - - -
7. Increased motor activity	- - - -	- - - -	- - - -
8. Loss of righting reflex	- - - -	- - - -	- - - -
9. Temperature	- - - -	- - - -	- - - -
10. Sedation	- - - -	- - - -	- - - -
11. Muscle relaxation	- - - -	- - - -	- - - -
12. Lacrimation & salivation	- - - -	- - - -	- - - -
13. Diarrhoea	- - - -	- - - -	- - - -

Different signs of acute toxicity were observed for all the animals after the drug administration. One animal from each standard & high dose group were found to be shown Straub reaction.

TABLE: 5.3 Clinical signs of acute toxicity:

Clinical signs	Group-I	Group-II	Group-III
Skin and fur	Normal	Normal	Normal
Eyes and mucous membranes	Normal	Normal	Normal
Respiratory systems	Normal	Normal	Normal
Circulatory system	Normal	Normal	Normal
Autonomic and central nervous system,	Normal	Normal	Normal
Somatomotor activity and Behaviour pattern	Normal	Normal	Normal

Clinical signs of toxicity were observed and they were found to be normal in all the animals of each group.

4. Individual Body weights:

TABLE: 5.4: Individual body weights

Groups	Body weight		
	DAY 0	DAY 7th	DAY 14th
Group-I	34.45±1.627	34.875±1.712	35.325±1.571
Group-II	33.6±1.010	33.825±0.900	34.125±0.920
Group-III	35.075±1.323	35.3±1.090	35.575±1.307

Number of animals=4; *p<0.05 is compared with control group, values are in MEAN±SEM.

All the animals weighed initially and on 7th & 14th day. In addition, weight recorded at the time of necropsy. There was no significant changes in body weight occur in all groups of animals.

4. Food intake:

The food intakes were measured initially and weekly thereafter during the period of treatment for all the animals. There was no significant changes in food intake occur in all mice.

5. Clinical Laboratory Investigations:

a) Haematology:

The blood was withdrawn from all animals by retro orbital puncture under light anesthesia on day 15 of the study and following haematological parameters were studied:

TABLE: 5.5 Hematological parameters in study animals

Haematological parameters	Group-I	Group-II	Group-III
Hemoglobin (g/ml)	14.15±0.132	14.05±0.155	14.2±0.227
Neutrophils (1000/mm³)	1.89±0.112	1.955±0.150	1.88±0.044
Lymphocytes (1000/mm³)	5.325±0.217	5.15±0.125	5.2375±0.179
Eosinophils (1000/mm³)	0.1725±0.006	0.1675±0.004	0.165±0.009
Monocytes (1000/mm³)	0.31±0.035	0.2925±0.012	0.2875±0.020
Basophils (1000/mm³)	0.0495±0.003	0.055±0.006	0.05275±0.004

Number of animals=4; *p<0.05 is compared with control group, values are in MEAN±SEM

There was no significant changes in haematological parameters occur in standard & double dose group as compared to control group.

b) Clinical Biochemistry:

The following biochemical parameters were studied by using semi auto analyzer.

TABLE: 5.6: Clinical biochemistry

Biochemical Parameters	Group-I (Distilled water)	Group-II (Alb400mg+ DEC300mg)	Group-III (Alb800mg+ DEC300mg)
Glucose	98.25±2.625	97.25±1.030	95.75±0.853
SGOT	34.5±2.11	35.1±0.99	34.9±4.3
SGPT	35.2±0.09	37.0±1.22	36±0.07
Creatinine	0.575±0.047	0.625±0.085	0.525±0.075
Serum cholesterol	113.32±12.33	112.12±12.35	113.11±12.29
HDL	81.05±5.3	80.54±5.4	82.00±5.0
Triglyceride	29.44±3.11	29.22±2.91	29.45±3.14
LDL	26.40±9.1	26.1±8.9	26.5±8.8
VLDL	5.77±0.82	5.9±0.62	5.82±0.66

Number of animals=4; *$p<0.05$ is compared with control group, values are in MEAN±SEM

There were no significant changes in biochemical parameters occur in standard & double dose group as compared to control group.

6. Pathology:

TABLE: 5.7: Necropsy & Organ Weights:

Organ Weights (gm)	Group-I	Group-II	Group-III
Liver	1.23±1.22	1.46±1.24	1.32±1.29
Kidney	0.20±2.0	0.22±2.11	0.22±2.24
Spleen	0.06±1.41	0.06±1.54	0.07±1.2
Heart	0.16±1.55	0.20±1.9	0.15±1.57

Number of animals=4; *$p<0.05$ is compared with control group, values are in MEAN±SEM

All the animals surviving at the end of treatment were sacrificed by cervical dislocation process. The animals were dissected and examined for gross lesions in different organs. There were no lesions found in any of above organ of animals. Different organs from all animals dissected free of fat and weights recorded as above. There were no significant changes occur in weights of all organs of different group animals.

DISCUSSION:

Our aim was to ascertain to what extent the safety & acceptability of high/low dose of albendazole with DEC in microfilaraemic individual by single dose oral administration had achieved. The people interviewed were of the age range 18 to 45 years. Males interviewed exceeded females in most of the localities. The question of drug compliance was most important and the study indicated better acceptability to the modified regimen. Although the study participants may not be very particular with details, such as the name of the drugs, it is more important that the people would receive and ingest the drugs to achieve the desired outcome of increased coverage supporting the goal of the programme.

Most of the study participants refused to take the albendazole in the form of chewable tablets & also they had no problem regarding swallowing the tablets. Thus it may not be mandatory to supply these tablets in the chewable form for the programme. The majority of study participants expressed that the programme was beneficial to them. Few of them had heard about MDA which indicated that awareness among them was less. There were also some subjects who refused to the use of net / coil for the prevention of mosquitoes.

Another observation is that swallowing of albendazole tablets was not difficult; so preparing DEC 300mg strength tablets can also reduce the number of tablets to be swallowed and it may also reduce the cost of the drug. Making albendazole tablets in non chewable formulation may also reduce the cost of the drug, which matters when it is introduced in large scale at the country level. All these information may help the programme when an alternative regimen will be planned for implementation.

Though this is not a community based study done in large scale, the pilot observation can be used in designing further studies in a community trial fashion to address the issue.

The observation of the study has indicated that if the high dose Albendazole (800mg) arm was found superior than low dose (400mg) arm in mf clearance or adult worm clearance; hence application of this dose schedule to the individuals will be safe & acceptable.

The study of toxic effect in mice has indicated that Albendazole & DEC are safe in mice in all respect at definite dose i.e. at 400 & 800mg of that human dose having no signs of toxicity.

As high dose of Albendazole with DEC found safe & not having any toxic effect in mice and also having safety & acceptability in micrifilaraemic individuals, hence this dose schedule is applicable.

CONCLUSION:

From the above work, it was concluded that this programme was safe & acceptable to the majority of the study participants. The responses from male as sex wise were good as compared to female subjects. Most of the subjects were preferred to take medicine in less frequent dose. They were not having any problem regarding characteristics of tablets. Also most of them were refused to take the chewable one. From this study, it was found a more effective regimen in reducing microfilaria and/or adult worm load, which was useful for maintaining persistent amicrofilaraemic state for a prolonged period. This regimen when applied to the global programme can effectively sustain the transmission blocking potential of the drug and thereby reducing the time required for elimination of the infection.

References

1) Bhaskar C, Harinath, Reddy MVR. Filariasis in India. Journal International Medical Science Academy 2000; 13:8-12.

2) Sabesan S, Palaniyandi M, Das PK, Michael E. Mapping of lymphatic filariasis in India. Ann Trop Med Parasitol 2000; 94:591-606.

3) ICMR. Prospects of eliminating lymphatic filariasis in India. ICMR Bulletin 2002; 32: 1- 14.

4) Ottesen EA, Duke BO, Karam M, Behbehani. Strategies and tools for the control /elimination of lymphatic filariasis. Bull World Health Organ 1997; 75: 491-503.

5) WHO. Lymphatic filariasis: progress of disability prevention activities. Weekly epidemiological record 2004; 79:417-24.

6) Preface. Elimination of lymphatic filariasis: a public-health challenge. Annals of Tropical Medicine & Parasitology 2002; 96: 3–13.

7) Ramaih KD, Das PK. Mass drug administration to eliminate lymphatic filariasis in India. Trend Parasitol 2004; 20:499-522.

8) Govt of India. Problems and elimination of lymphatic filariasis in India. National vector borne diseases control program, Ministry of Health and Family Welfare. (Cited 2005 May14).

9) Park K. Parks Textbook of Preventive and Social medicine. 18th ed. Jabalpur: Banarsidas Bhanot, 2005.

10) Shenoy RK, Sandhya K, Suma TK, Kumaraswami V. A preliminary study of filariasis related acute adenolymphangitis with special reference to precipitating factors and treatment modalities. SE Asian J Trop Med Pub Hlth 1995; 26:301–5.

11) Weil GJ, Lammie PJ, Weiss N. The ICT filariasis test: a rapid format antigen test of diagnosis of Bancroftian filariasis. Parasitol Today 1997; 13:401–4.

12) WHO. National Filariasis Control Programme in India and New Strategies for Its Control. (Cited 2005 May14).

13) Ramaiah KD, Vijay KN, Chandrakala AV, Augustin DJ Appavoo NC, Das PK. Effectiveness of community and health services-organized drug delivery strategies for elimination of lymphatic filariasis in rural areas of Tamil Nadu, India .Tropical Medicine and International Health 2001; 6 : 1062-9.

14) Chakroborty .P,Text book of Medical Parasitology.

15) Paniker, Text book of Medical Parasitology.

16) Chatterjee K.D.Parasitology.

17) Hardmann Joe G, Limbird, and Goodman Gilman AlFred, The pharmacological basis of therapeutic.

18) Molyneux D. Lymphatic Filariasis (Elephantiasis) Elimination: A public health success and development opportunity. Filaria Journal 2003; 2: 13.

19) Molyneux DH, Zagaria N. Lymphatic filariasis elimination: progress in global programme development. Annals of Tropical Medicine & Parasitology 2002; 96 (2 Suppl): 15S–40S.

20) Ramaiah KD, Vijay Kumar KN, Ravi R, Das PK. Situation analysis in a large urban area of India, prior to launching a programme of mass drug administration to eliminate lymphatic filariasis. Ann Trop Med Parasitol 2005; 99; 243-5.

21) Charles H W, Radday J, Thomas G Streit, et al. Spatial clustering of filarial transmission before and after a Mass Drug Administration in a setting of low infection prevalence .Filaria Journal 2004;3:3.

22) Simonsen PE, Meyrowitsch DW, Mukoko DA, et al. The effect of repeated half-yearly diethylcarbamazine mass treatment on *wuchereria bancrofti* infection and transmission in two east African communities with different levels of endemicity. Am J Trop Med Hyg 2004; 70: 63.

23) Brabin L. Sex differentials in susceptibility to lymphatic filariasis and implications for maternal child immunity.*Epidemiol Infect* 1990; 105: 335-53.

24) Dash AP, Mohapata N, Hazra RK, Acharya AS. Transmission dynamics of filariasis in Khurda district of Orissa, India. *Southeast Asian J Trop Med Public Health* 1998; 29: 137-40.

25) Evans DB, Gelband H, Binka FN. Social and economic factors and the control of lymphatic filariasis: a review. *Acta Trop* 1993; 53: 1-26.

26) Kar SK, Mania J, Kar PK. Prevalence of lymphatic nodules in a bancroftian endemic population. *Acta Trop* 1993; 55: 53-60.

27) Kumar A, Dash AP, Mansing GD. Prevalence of filariasis in rural Puri, Orissa. *J Commun Dis* 1994; 26: 215-20.

28) Kumar A. Human filariasis: infection rate as the uniform measurable criterion for filarial endemicity. *J Commun Dis* 1996; 28: 163-7.

29) Kumaraswami V. The clinical manifestations of lymphatic filariasis, In: TB Nutman, ed. Lymphatic Filariasis. London: Imperial College Press, 2000: 103-25.

30) Michael E, Bundy DAP, Grenfell BT. Re-assessing the global prevalence and distribution of lymphatic filariasis. *Parasitology* 1996; 112: 409-28.

31) Pani SP, Balakrishnan N, Srividya A, Bundy DAP, Grenfell BT. Clinical epidemiology of bancroftian filariasis: effect of age and gender. *Trans R Soc Trop Med Hyg* 1991; 85: 260-4.

32) Partono F. The spectrum of disease in lymphatic filariasis, In: Filariasis. *Ciba Found Sympos* 1987; 127: 15-31.

33) Ramaiah KD, Ramu K, Vijaykumar KN, Guyatt H 1996. Epidemiology of acute filarial episodes caused by *Wuchereria bancrofti* infection in two rural villages in Tamil Nadu, South India. *Trans R Soc Trop Med Hyg* 1996; 90: 639.

34) Ramaiah KD, Das PK, Michael E, Guyatt H. The economic burden of lymphatic filariasis in India. *Parasitol Today* 2000; 16: 251-3.

35) Rath RN, Das RK, Mishara G, Mohapatra BN, Ramakrishna C. Bancroftian filariasis in two rural selected communities – A comparative study of filariometric data. *J Commun Dis* 1984; 16: 104-22.

36) Sharma RVSN, Vallishayee RS, Mayurnath S, Narayanan PR, Radhamani MP, Tripathy SP.Prevalence survey of filariasis in two villages in Chingleput district of Tamil Nadu. *Indian J Med Res* 1987; 85: 522-30.

37) Sharma S, Sharma M, Rathur S. Bancroftian filariasis in the Varanasi region of north India: an epidemiological study. *Ann Trop Med Parasitol* 1999; 93: 379-87.

38) Ottesen EA, Duke BOL, Karam M, Behbehani K: Strategies and tools for the control/elimination of lymphatic filariasis. *Bull World Health Organ* 1997, 75:491-503

39) Sabesan S, Palaniyandi M, Das PK, Michael E: Mapping of lymphatic filariasis in India. *Ann Trop Med Parasitol* 2000, 94:591-606

40) Das PK, Pani SP: "Filariasis", Epidemiology and control. *In: Helminthology in India (Edited by: Prof ML Sood)* 2002

41) Das PK, Ramaiah KD, Augusstin DJ, Kumar A: Towards Elimination Of lymphatic filariasis in India. *Trends Parasitol* 2001, 17:457-460

42) Das PK, Pani SP: Towards elimination of lymphatic filariasis in India: Problems, challenges, opportunities and new initiatives. *J Int Med Sci Acad* 2000, 13:18-26

43) Das PK, Pani SP, Krishnamurthy K: Prospects of elimination of lymphatic filariasis in India. *ICMR Bulletin* 2002

44) Reddy GS, Vengatesvarlou N, Das PK, Vanamail P, Vijayan AP, Sasikala K, Pani SP: Tolerability and efficacy of single-dose diethyl carbamazine (DEC) or ivermectin in the clearance of Wuchereria bancrofti microfilaraemia in Pondicherry, south India. *Trop Med Int Health* 2000, 5:779-785

45) World Medical Association: Declaration of Helsinki – Recommendations guiding physicians in biomedical research involving human subjects. *In: WHO Technical Report Series, No. 850, Annex 3* 1995, 30-33

46) World Health Organization: Guidelines for good clinical practice (GCP) for trials on pharmaceutical products. *WHO Technical Report Series, No. 850, Annex 3* 1995, 1-35

47) Indian Council of Medical Research: Statement of general principles on ethical considerations involving human subjects In: *Ethical guidelines for biomedical research on human subjects.* 2000, 1-8

48) Addiss DG, Beach MJ, Streit TG, Lutwic S, LeConte FH, Lafontant JG, Hightower AW, Lammie PJ: Randomized placebo-controlled comparison of ivermectin and albendazole alone and in combination for Wuchereria bancrofti microfilaraemia in Haitian children. *Lancet* 1997, 350:480-484

49) Beach MJ, Streit TG, Addiss DG, Prospere R, Roberts JM, Lammie PJ: Assessment of combined ivermectin and albendazole for treatment of intestinal helminth and Wuchereria bancrofti infections in Haitian school children. *Am J Trop Med Hyg* 1999, 60:479-486

50) Dunyo SK, Nkrumah FK, Simonsen PE: A randomized doubleblind placebo-controlled field trial of ivermectin and albendazole alone and in combination for the treatment of lymphatic filariasis in Ghana. *Trans R Soc Trop Med Hyg* 2000, 94:205- 211

51) Ismail MM, Jayakodi RL, Weil CJ, Nirmalan N, Jayasinghe KSA, Abeyewickrema W, Rezvi Sheriff MH, Rajaratnam HN, Amarasekara N, DeSilva DCL, *et al*: Efficacy of single dose combinations of Albendazole, ivermectin and diethylcarbamazine citrate for the treatment of bancroftian filariasis. *Trans R Soc Trop Med Hyg* 1998, 92:94-97

52) Horton J, Witt C, Ottesen EA, Lazdins JK, Addiss DG, Awadzi K, Beach MJ, Belizario VY, Dunyo SK, Espinel M, *et al*: An analysis of the safety of the single dose, two drug regimens used in programmes to eliminate lymphatic filariasis. *Parasitology* 2000, 121:S147-S160

53) Ghosh, M. N., Toxicity studies. In *Fundamentals of Experimental Pharmacology*, Scientific Book Agency, Calcutta, pp. 190–195.

54) Paget, G. E. and Barnes, J. M., Toxicity tests. In *Evaluation of Drug Activities: Pharmacometrics* (eds Lawrence, D. R. and Bacharach,A. L.), Academic Press, London, 1964, pp. 140–161.

55) Turner, R., Acute toxicity: The determination of LD50. In *Screening Methods in Pharmacology*, Academic Press, New York, 1965, pp.300.

56) Turner, R., Quantal responses. Calculation of ED50. In *Screening Methods in Pharmacology*, Academic Press, New York, 1965, pp.61–63.

57) Lorke, D., A new approach to practical acute toxicity testing. *Arch. Toxicol.*, 1983, **53**, 275–289.

58) Akah, P. A., Ezike, A. C., Nwafor, S. V., Okoli, C. O. and Enwerem, N. M., Evaluation of the antiasthmatic property of *Acystasia gangetica* leaf extracts. *J. Ethnopharmacol.*, 2003, **89**, 25–36.

59) Osadebe, P. O. and Okoye, F. B. C., Antiinflammatory effects of crude methanolic extract and fractions of *Alchornea cordifolia* leaves. *J. Ethnopharmacol.*, 2003, **89**, 19–24.

60) F inney, D J (1971) Probit Analysis, Cambridge U niver sity Pr ess , Cambr idge, U.K.

61) British Toxicology Society (1984) Special report: a new approach to the classification of substances and preparations on the basis of their acute toxicity, Human Toxicol., 3:85-92.

62) Van den Heuval, M J, A D Dayan and R O Shillaker (1987). Evaluation of the BTS approach to the testing of substances and preparations for their acute toxicity,Human Toxicol., 6:279-291.

63) Van den Heuvel, M J, D G Clark, R J Fielder, P P Koundakjian, G J A Oliver, D Pelling, N J Tomlinson, and A P Walker (1990). The international validation of a fixed-dose procedure as an alternative to the classical LD50 test, Fd. Chem. Toxicol., 28:469-482.

64) Whitehead, A and R N Curnow (1992). Statistical evaluation of the fixed-dose procedure, Fd. Chem. Toxic., 30:313-324.

65) Stallard N and A Whitehead (1995). Reducing numbers in the fixed-dose procedure, Human Expt. Toxicol., 14:315-323.

66) Lipnick, R L, J A Cotruvo, R N Hill, R D Bruce, K A Stitzel, A P Walker, I Chu, M Goddard, L Segal, J A Springer, and R C Myers (1995). *Comparison of the Up-and-Down, Conventional LD50, and Fixed-Dose Acute Toxicity Procedures.* Fd Chem. Toxic. 33: 223-231.

67) Yam, J, P J Reer, and R D Bruce (1991). *Comparison of the Up-and-Down Method and the Fixed-Dose Procedure for Acute Oral Toxicity Testing.* Fd Chem. Toxic. 29:259-263.

68) Diener, W; U Mischke, E Schlede and D Kayser (1995). *The biometric evaluation of the OECD modified version of the acute toxic class method (oral).* Arch.Toxicol. 69: 729-734.

69) Diener, W; and E Schlede. (1996). *Brief an den Herausgeber: ML Prinzip und ATCMethode.* ALTEX 13(4): 238-239.

70) Diener, W; and E Schlede (1996). *Letter to the Editor: FDP and ATC method: a mathematical comparison.* Human Experim.Toxicol. 15: 855-856.

71) Diener, W; L Siccha, U Mischke, D Kayser and E Schlede (1994*). The biometric evaluation of the acute-toxic-class method (oral).* Arch.Toxicol. 68: 599-610.

72) Schlede, E; U Mischke, W Diener and D Kayser. (1995). *The international validation study of the acute-toxic-class method (oral).* Arch.Toxicol. 69: 659-670.

73) Dixon, W J, and A M Mood (1948). A method for obtaining and analyzing sensitivity data. J. Amer. Statist. Assoc. 43:109-126. *Appendix O-1 Up-and-Down Procedure Peer Panel Report* O-12 K. Stitzel and G. Carr - 03/18/1999

74) Dixon, W J (1991). Staircase Bioassay: The Up-and-Down Method. Neurosci. Biobehav. Rev. 15:47-50.

75) Brownlee, K A, J L Hodges, Jr., and M Rosenblatt (1953). J Amer. Stat. Assoc., 48:262-277.

76) Hsi, B P (1969). J Amer. Stat. Assoc., 64:147-162.

77) Dixon, W J and Dixon Statistical Associates (1991). Design and Analysis of Quantal Dose Response Experiments (with Emphasis on Staircase Designs).

78) Bruce, R D (1985). An up-and-down procedure for acute toxicity testing. Fundam. Appl. Tox., 5:151-157.

79) ASTM (1987) E 1163-87, Standard test method for estimating acute oral toxicity in rats. American Society for Testing Materials, Philadelphia PA, USA.

80) Dixon, W J (1965). The up-and down method for small samples. J. Amer. Statist. Assoc., 60:967-978.

81) Finney, D J (1971). Probit Analysis, 3rd ed., Cambridge University Press, Cambridge, England, 50-80.

82) Stallard, N and A Whitehead (1996). A preliminary statistical evaluation of the up-and down procedure. Medical and Pharmaceutical Research Unit, University of Reading.

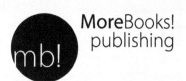
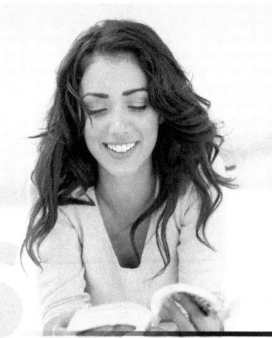

Printed in the USA
CPSIA information can be obtained
at www.ICGtesting.com
LVHW082153290124
770308LV00023B/190